self care

A Journal to Reclaim Your Time to Rest and Rejuvenate

chartwell
books

Contents

Tuning into Your Needs

Time Management

Cycle of Celebration

Self Love

Write it Out

Tuning into Your Needs

Y ou were put on this earth to live a radically fulfilling, purpose-driven, joyful life. You are worthy of this kind of life. You deserve to wake up each day with excitement coursing through your body and spirit in anticipation for what lies ahead.

Unfortunately, this kind of life is elusive for many. In our distracting, fast-paced, and demanding world, it can be easy to put yourself last. You may find yourself putting your needs at the bottom of your ever-growing to-do list. Maybe you actively prioritize the needs of everyone else above your own. Perhaps you're depleted at the end of the day, exhausted from trying to satisfy everyone else but yourself.

Many of us struggle with how much attention and care we need to give to ourselves, and we often allot much less than what we actually require. This overextension and underestimation of needs can lead to feeling burnt out, and like you have no control in your own life. Reaching for things we want (rather than the bare minimum we need to survive) and providing ourselves with more than time and space can help us feel like more active participants in our own lives.

By becoming aware of your surroundings, working to process difficult emotions, building healthy boundaries, and then pursuing the things that make your soul sing, you can apply these methods of self care to course-correct a life that feels out of hand.

Five Senses Exercise

These simple exercises can be done anytime and anywhere to bring you firmly into the experience of your present moment. By recognizing your five senses, which are working all the time even if you don't notice them, you acknowledge your present experience. It is this acknowledgment that brings your consciousness back to here and now.

Ask yourself the following questions and respond in your mind. Or, if you're somewhere private, you can say your answers out loud. Do this exercise daily. If you find yourself feeling stuck in the past or the future, repeat this exercise numerous times a day until staying in the moment becomes a habit.

Below is the small, daily exercise that you can practice to ground yourself.

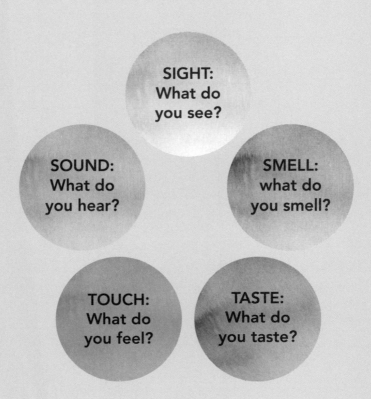

SIGHT:
What do
you see?

SOUND:
What do
you hear?

SMELL:
what do
you smell?

TOUCH:
What do
you feel?

TASTE:
What do
you taste?

Sound

If you close your eyes, what are some of the quieter noises you can perceive?

_____

_____

_____

_____

_____

What is the loudest sound you hear?

_____

_____

_____

_____

_____

Sight

What in your current setting draws the eye the most?

_____

_____

_____

_____

_____

_____

_____

What do you see in the periphery of your vision?

_____

_____

_____

_____

_____

_____

_____

Smell

Describe the strongest aroma currently in your vicinity.

_____

_____

_____

_____

_____

_____

What memories does this smell bring up?

_____

_____

_____

_____

_____

_____

Taste

After eating something, take a few extra minutes to chew it over and savor the flavor.
Do you discover any additional flavors?

_____

_____

_____

_____

_____

_____

How would you describe the absence of taste?

_____

_____

_____

_____

_____

_____

_____

Touch

Scan your body from head-to-toe. What are the most prominent physical sensations that you feel?

_____

_____

_____

_____

_____

_____

_____

Which areas of your body feel most sensitive to you?

_____

_____

_____

_____

_____

_____

_____

Identifying Your Boundaries

On the left-hand side of the following pages, make a list of all of the things in your life that *make you feel safe*. There's no right or wrong entries seeing as this list is unique to you.

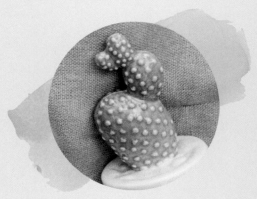

Examples include:

- Your favorite people who make you feel emotionally safe.
- A movie that gets you to your "good place."
- A song or genre that resonates with you.
- Types of clothing that you like to wear.
- An amount of money that makes you feel financially secure.
- The kind of home or shelter that makes you feel safe.
- Free time that lets you be yourself.

On the right-hand side, make a list of all of the things in your life that *make you feel unsafe*. This side may be emotionally difficult to write.

You can include:

- Traumas
- Things that make you feel disrespected
- Things you don't like
- Values that go against your own
- Include anything that threatens your sense of self on this list.
- Situations that make you uncomfortable

When you assess these lists side-by-side, the boundaries that suit your life should become clear. Fill in the boundaries you discover in the bottom section on boundaries.

For example:

You wrote that your home makes you feel secure on the SAFE side. On the UNSAFE side, you wrote that you don't feel safe when someone drops by your home announced. One of your boundaries would be: "I need people to give me advance notice." Then, find ways to enforce that boundary, in this case by letting people know the amount of notice you need.

Home

SAFE

UNSAFE

BOUNDARIES

Work

BOUNDARIES

Social

SAFE

_____

_____

_____

_____

_____

UNSAFE

_____

_____

_____

_____

_____

BOUNDARIES

_____

_____

_____

_____

_____

_____

_____

Journal Therapy

An important part of self care is discussing issues (large and small) with a mental health professional that can unapologetically provide hard truths, or tell you to be kinder to yourself. Keeping a log of what you talk about in therapy and how it makes you feel can help you get the most out of your mental health professional.

If you aren't in therapy, you might want to consider it eventually, but you can also use these pages to try and work out issues that are giving you a hard time.

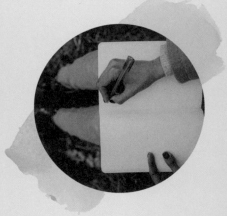

Before Therapy

Date	Month	Year

Issues you wanted to talk about:

Triggering events of the week:

_____

_____

_____

_____

_____

_____

Things you're working on:

_____

_____

_____

_____

_____

_____

After Therapy

Things discussed:

How are you processing these feelings?

Do any specific memories arise?

Before Therapy

Date	Month	Year

Issues you wanted to talk about:

Triggering events of the week:

_____

_____

_____

_____

_____

_____

_____

Things you're working on:

_____

_____

_____

_____

_____

_____

_____

After Therapy

Things discussed:

_____

_____

_____

_____

_____

_____

_____

_____

_____

_____

_____

_____

_____

_____

How are you processing these feelings?

_____

_____

_____

_____

_____

_____

_____

Do any specific memories arise?

_____

_____

_____

_____

_____

_____

_____

_____

Before Therapy

Issues you wanted to talk about:

Triggering events of the week:

_____

_____

_____

_____

_____

_____

_____

Things you're working on:

_____

_____

_____

_____

_____

_____

_____

After Therapy

Things discussed:

_____

_____

_____

_____

_____

_____

_____

_____

_____

_____

_____

_____

_____

_____

_____

_____

How are you processing these feelings?

_____

_____

_____

_____

_____

_____

_____

Do any specific memories arise?

_____

_____

_____

_____

_____

_____

_____

_____

Manifesting Goals

Manifestation is using your energy, belief system, thoughts, and visualization to bring an idea into your physical reality. In practice, manifestation takes time and a lot of thought to bring into action. Fill out the prompts in order below to help yourself get the hang of bringing what you want into the fold.

I WANT:

What are some opportunities in your life that reflect this manifestation?

What are some actions you can take to harness those opportunities?

Imagine the details:

Paint yourself into the picture:

What are some ways you can make it more real in your mind?

How much do you believe it?

List some affirmations to help you manifest your goal: (think 'I am' statements)

How did it pan out?

I WANT:

What are some opportunities in your life that reflect this manifestation?

What are some actions you can take to harness those opportunities?

Imagine the details:

Paint yourself into the picture:

What are some ways you can make it more real in your mind?

How much do you believe it?

List some affirmations to help you manifest your goal: (think 'I am' statements)

How did it pan out?

I WANT:

What are some opportunities in your life that reflect this manifestation?

What are some actions you can take to harness those opportunities?

Imagine the details:

Paint yourself into the picture:

What are some ways you can
make it more real in your mind?

How much do you believe it?

List some affirmations to help you
manifest your goal: (think 'I am' statements)

How did it pan out?

I WANT:

What are some opportunities in your life that reflect this manifestation?

What are some actions you can take to harness those opportunities?

Imagine the details:

Paint yourself into the picture:

What are some ways you can make it more real in your mind?

How much do you believe it?

List some affirmations to help you manifest your goal: (think 'I am' statements)

How did it pan out?

I WANT:

What are some opportunities in your life that reflect this manifestation?

What are some actions you can take to harness those opportunities?

Imagine the details:

Paint yourself into the picture:

What are some ways you can
make it more real in your mind?

How much do you believe it?

List some affirmations to help you
manifest your goal: (think 'I am' statements)

How did it pan out?

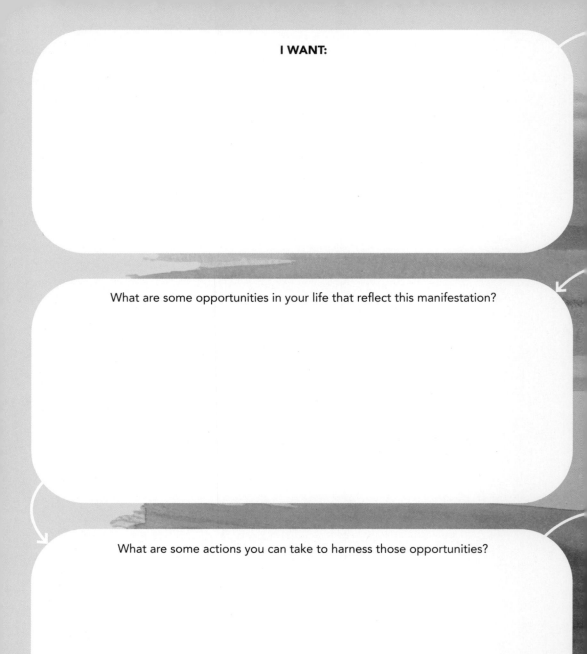

I WANT:

What are some opportunities in your life that reflect this manifestation?

What are some actions you can take to harness those opportunities?

Imagine the details:

Paint yourself into the picture:

What are some ways you can
make it more real in your mind?

How much do you believe it?

List some affirmations to help you
manifest your goal: (think 'I am' statements)

How did it pan out?

Creating a Vision Board

Create a vision board to serve as a reminder of the life you're working to manifest.

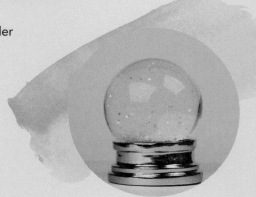

You'll need:

Music that makes you feel inspired

Scissors

Magazines

Writing utensil

A glue stick or tape

1. Play inspiring music and sit for five minutes with your eyes closed. Imagine—in vivid detail—the things that would bring you the most joy.

2. Open your eyes and begin filling in the details in the following journal pages.

3. Flip through the magazines and cut out photos and words that fit the vision you imagined.

4. Once you've cut out several images and words, attach them to the following journal entries.

Describe:

Your day-to-day routine:

_____

_____

_____

_____

_____

_____

Your career:

_____

_____

_____

_____

Your love life:

_____

_____

_____

_____

Your social life:

_____

_____

_____

_____

Your wardrobe:

_____

_____

_____

_____

_____

_____

Your mood:

_____

_____

_____

_____

_____

_____

Your home:

_____

_____

_____

_____

_____

_____

Your favorite breakfast:

_____

_____

_____

_____

_____

_____

One quirky thing you always have on you:

_____

_____

_____

_____

_____

_____

How you spend your free time:

_____

_____

_____

_____

_____

_____

What do you spurge on:

_____

_____

_____

_____

_____

_____

A weekly activity you never miss:

_____

_____

_____

_____

_____

_____

Describe:

Your day-to-day routine:

_____

_____

_____

Your career:

_____

_____

_____

_____

Your love life:

_____

_____

_____

_____

Your social life:

Your wardrobe:

Your mood:

Your home:

_____

_____

_____

_____

Your favorite breakfast:

_____

_____

_____

_____

One quirky thing you always have on you:

_____

_____

_____

_____

How you spend your free time:

_____

_____

_____

_____

What do you spurge on:

_____

_____

_____

_____

A weekly activity you never miss:

_____

_____

_____

_____

Describe:

Your day-to-day routine:

Your career:

Your love life:

Your social life:

_____

_____

_____

_____

Your wardrobe:

_____

_____

_____

_____

Your mood:

_____

_____

_____

_____

Your home:

_____

_____

_____

_____

Your favorite breakfast:

_____

_____

_____

_____

One quirky thing you always have on you:

_____

_____

_____

_____

How you spend your free time:

_____

_____

_____

_____

What do you spurge on:

_____

_____

_____

_____

A weekly activity you never miss:

_____

_____

_____

_____

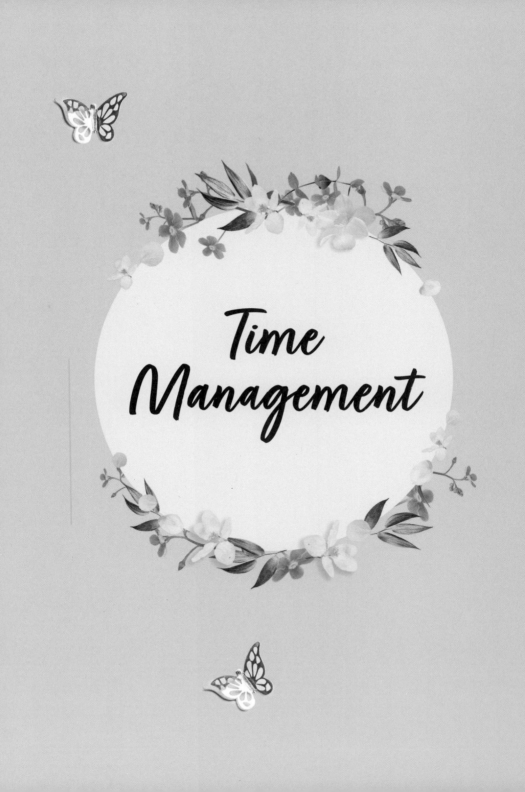

Time Management

Your time is precious. Once you've identified the general ebb and flow of your energy, you can then schedule your day for maximum efficiency and happiness. By placing high-priority and engaging tasks during your periods of high energy and low-priority or uninteresting tasks during your periods of low energy, you can create a time management system that works with your natural energy cycle. This system is called time blocking.

Blocking out your time helps you manage your priorities and prevent burnout. Use the following pages to learn about how you interact with time and build out your time blocking practice. It is important that you prioritize self care when time blocking your day. Self care exercises help keep you stable, happy, and balanced, which will make your day even more productive and efficient. Scheduling in breaks, allowing yourself to do "nothing" as an activity (you deserve some downtime to recharge!), and prioritizing time blocks for fun and rejuvenation will create balance and joy in your life.

To effectively time block, you need to employ time integrity. Set aside an amount of time for a task and stick to it—giving all of your focus to only that task during a specified period of time. You can use your phone or a time cube to keep track of time. A time cube is a tabletop timer broken down into time increments of five, fifteen, thirty, and sixty minutes. This helps you mentally turn a task into a kind of beat-the-clock game.

Morning Pages

Complete these pages as soon as
you wake up every day for a week.

Date	Month	Year

M   T   W   TH   F   SA   SU

Thoughts:

_____

_____

_____

To be completed:

☐ _____   ☐ _____

☐ _____   ☐ _____

☐ _____   ☐ _____

Intention:

_____

_____

_____

Gratitude: **Dreams:**

1 _____   1 _____

2 _____   2 _____

3 _____   3 _____

Date	Month	Year		M	T	W	TH	F	SA	SU

Thoughts:

_____

_____

_____

_____

To be completed:

☐ _____   ☐ _____

☐ _____   ☐ _____

☐ _____   ☐ _____

Intention:

_____

_____

_____

Gratitude: Dreams:

1 _____   1 _____

2 _____   2 _____

3 _____   3 _____

MORNING PAGES

| Date | Month | Year | M | T | W | TH | F | SA | SU |

Thoughts:

_____

_____

_____

_____

To be completed:

☐ _____   ☐ _____

☐ _____   ☐ _____

☐ _____   ☐ _____

Intention:

_____

_____

_____

Gratitude: Dreams:

1 _____   1 _____

2 _____   2 _____

3 _____   3 _____

Date	Month	Year	M	T	W	TH	F	SA	SU

Thoughts:

To be completed:

☐ _____   ☐ _____

☐ _____   ☐ _____

☐ _____   ☐ _____

Intention:

Gratitude: Dreams:

1 _____   1 _____

2 _____   2 _____

3 _____   3 _____

MORNING PAGES

Date	Month	Year	M	T	W	TH	F	SA	SU

Thoughts:

_____

_____

_____

_____

To be completed:

☐ _____   ☐ _____

☐ _____   ☐ _____

☐ _____   ☐ _____

Intention:

_____

_____

_____

Gratitude: Dreams:

1 _____   1 _____

2 _____   2 _____

3 _____   3 _____

Date	Month	Year	M	T	W	TH	F	SA	SU

Thoughts:

To be completed:

☐ _____   ☐ _____

☐ _____   ☐ _____

☐ _____   ☐ _____

Intention:

Gratitude:

1 _____

2 _____

3 _____

Dreams:

1 _____

2 _____

3 _____

MORNING PAGES

Date	Month	Year	M	T	W	TH	F	SA	SU

Thoughts:

_____

_____

_____

_____

To be completed:

☐ _____   ☐ _____

☐ _____   ☐ _____

☐ _____   ☐ _____

Intention:

_____

_____

_____

Gratitude: **Dreams:**

1 _____   1 _____

2 _____   2 _____

3 _____   3 _____

| Date | Month | Year | M | T | W | TH | F | SA | SU |

Thoughts:

To be completed:

☐ _____   ☐ _____

☐ _____   ☐ _____

☐ _____   ☐ _____

Intention:

Gratitude: Dreams:

1 _____   1 _____

2 _____   2 _____

3 _____   3 _____

Keeping Track of Your Time

To figure out your general flow, you must be in sync with your unique rhythms. This simple, week-long exercise will tell you a lot about yourself and how to schedule your day.

TIME	ACTIVITY	PRODUCTIVITY	MOOD TRACKER
6:00 a.m.		− ☐ ☐ +	
7:00 a.m.		− ☐ ☐ +	
8:00 a.m.		− ☐ ☐ +	
9:00 a.m.		− ☐ ☐ +	
10:00 a.m.		− ☐ ☐ +	
11:00 a.m.		− ☐ ☐ +	
12:00 p.m.		− ☐ ☐ +	
1:00 p.m.		− ☐ ☐ +	
2:00 p.m.		− ☐ ☐ +	
3:00 p.m.		− ☐ ☐ +	
4:00 p.m.		− ☐ ☐ +	
5:00 p.m.		− ☐ ☐ +	
6:00 p.m.		− ☐ ☐ +	
7:00 p.m.		− ☐ ☐ +	
8:00 p.m.		− ☐ ☐ +	
9:00 p.m.		− ☐ ☐ +	
10:00 p.m.		− ☐ ☐ +	

TIME	ACTIVITY	PRODUCTIVITY	MOOD TRACKER
6:00 a.m.		− ☐ ☐ +	
7:00 a.m.		− ☐ ☐ +	
8:00 a.m.		− ☐ ☐ +	
9:00 a.m.		− ☐ ☐ +	
10:00 a.m.		− ☐ ☐ +	
11:00 a.m.		− ☐ ☐ +	
12:00 p.m.		− ☐ ☐ +	
1:00 p.m.		− ☐ ☐ +	
2:00 p.m.		− ☐ ☐ +	
3:00 p.m.		− ☐ ☐ +	
4:00 p.m.		− ☐ ☐ +	
5:00 p.m.		− ☐ ☐ +	
6:00 p.m.		− ☐ ☐ +	
7:00 p.m.		− ☐ ☐ +	
8:00 p.m.		− ☐ ☐ +	
9:00 p.m.		− ☐ ☐ +	
10:00 p.m.		− ☐ ☐ +	

KEEPING TRACK OF YOUR TIME

TIME	ACTIVITY	PRODUCTIVITY	MOOD TRACKER
6:00 a.m.		− ☐ ☐ +	
7:00 a.m.		− ☐ ☐ +	
8:00 a.m.		− ☐ ☐ +	
9:00 a.m.		− ☐ ☐ +	
10:00 a.m.		− ☐ ☐ +	
11:00 a.m.		− ☐ ☐ +	
12:00 p.m.		− ☐ ☐ +	
1:00 p.m.		− ☐ ☐ +	
2:00 p.m.		− ☐ ☐ +	
3:00 p.m.		− ☐ ☐ +	
4:00 p.m.		− ☐ ☐ +	
5:00 p.m.		− ☐ ☐ +	
6:00 p.m.		− ☐ ☐ +	
7:00 p.m.		− ☐ ☐ +	
8:00 p.m.		− ☐ ☐ +	
9:00 p.m.		− ☐ ☐ +	
10:00 p.m.		− ☐ ☐ +	

TIME	ACTIVITY	PRODUCTIVITY	MOOD TRACKER
6:00 a.m.		− ☐ ☐ +	
7:00 a.m.		− ☐ ☐ +	
8:00 a.m.		− ☐ ☐ +	
9:00 a.m.		− ☐ ☐ +	
10:00 a.m.		− ☐ ☐ +	
11:00 a.m.		− ☐ ☐ +	
12:00 p.m.		− ☐ ☐ +	
1:00 p.m.		− ☐ ☐ +	
2:00 p.m.		− ☐ ☐ +	
3:00 p.m.		− ☐ ☐ +	
4:00 p.m.		− ☐ ☐ +	
5:00 p.m.		− ☐ ☐ +	
6:00 p.m.		− ☐ ☐ +	
7:00 p.m.		− ☐ ☐ +	
8:00 p.m.		− ☐ ☐ +	
9:00 p.m.		− ☐ ☐ +	
10:00 p.m.		− ☐ ☐ +	

KEEPING TRACK OF YOUR TIME

TIME	ACTIVITY	PRODUCTIVITY	MOOD TRACKER
6:00 a.m.		− ☐ ☐ +	
7:00 a.m.		− ☐ ☐ +	
8:00 a.m.		− ☐ ☐ +	
9:00 a.m.		− ☐ ☐ +	
10:00 a.m.		− ☐ ☐ +	
11:00 a.m.		− ☐ ☐ +	
12:00 p.m.		− ☐ ☐ +	
1:00 p.m.		− ☐ ☐ +	
2:00 p.m.		− ☐ ☐ +	
3:00 p.m.		− ☐ ☐ +	
4:00 p.m.		− ☐ ☐ +	
5:00 p.m.		− ☐ ☐ +	
6:00 p.m.		− ☐ ☐ +	
7:00 p.m.		− ☐ ☐ +	
8:00 p.m.		− ☐ ☐ +	
9:00 p.m.		− ☐ ☐ +	
10:00 p.m.		− ☐ ☐ +	

TIME	ACTIVITY	PRODUCTIVITY	MOOD TRACKER
6:00 a.m.		− ☐ ☐ +	
7:00 a.m.		− ☐ ☐ +	
8:00 a.m.		− ☐ ☐ +	
9:00 a.m.		− ☐ ☐ +	
10:00 a.m.		− ☐ ☐ +	
11:00 a.m.		− ☐ ☐ +	
12:00 p.m.		− ☐ ☐ +	
1:00 p.m.		− ☐ ☐ +	
2:00 p.m.		− ☐ ☐ +	
3:00 p.m.		− ☐ ☐ +	
4:00 p.m.		− ☐ ☐ +	
5:00 p.m.		− ☐ ☐ +	
6:00 p.m.		− ☐ ☐ +	
7:00 p.m.		− ☐ ☐ +	
8:00 p.m.		− ☐ ☐ +	
9:00 p.m.		− ☐ ☐ +	
10:00 p.m.		− ☐ ☐ +	

KEEPING TRACK OF YOUR TIME

TIME	ACTIVITY	PRODUCTIVITY	MOOD TRACKER
6:00 a.m.		− ☐ ☐ +	
7:00 a.m.		− ☐ ☐ +	
8:00 a.m.		− ☐ ☐ +	
9:00 a.m.		− ☐ ☐ +	
10:00 a.m.		− ☐ ☐ +	
11:00 a.m.		− ☐ ☐ +	
12:00 p.m.		− ☐ ☐ +	
1:00 p.m.		− ☐ ☐ +	
2:00 p.m.		− ☐ ☐ +	
3:00 p.m.		− ☐ ☐ +	
4:00 p.m.		− ☐ ☐ +	
5:00 p.m.		− ☐ ☐ +	
6:00 p.m.		− ☐ ☐ +	
7:00 p.m.		− ☐ ☐ +	
8:00 p.m.		− ☐ ☐ +	
9:00 p.m.		− ☐ ☐ +	
10:00 p.m.		− ☐ ☐ +	

TIME	ACTIVITY	PRODUCTIVITY	MOOD TRACKER
6:00 a.m.		− ☐ ☐ +	
7:00 a.m.		− ☐ ☐ +	
8:00 a.m.		− ☐ ☐ +	
9:00 a.m.		− ☐ ☐ +	
10:00 a.m.		− ☐ ☐ +	
11:00 a.m.		− ☐ ☐ +	
12:00 p.m.		− ☐ ☐ +	
1:00 p.m.		− ☐ ☐ +	
2:00 p.m.		− ☐ ☐ +	
3:00 p.m.		− ☐ ☐ +	
4:00 p.m.		− ☐ ☐ +	
5:00 p.m.		− ☐ ☐ +	
6:00 p.m.		− ☐ ☐ +	
7:00 p.m.		− ☐ ☐ +	
8:00 p.m.		− ☐ ☐ +	
9:00 p.m.		− ☐ ☐ +	
10:00 p.m.		− ☐ ☐ +	

KEEPING TRACK OF YOUR TIME

TIME	ACTIVITY	PRODUCTIVITY	MOOD TRACKER
6:00 a.m.		− ☐ ☐ +	
7:00 a.m.		− ☐ ☐ +	
8:00 a.m.		− ☐ ☐ +	
9:00 a.m.		− ☐ ☐ +	
10:00 a.m.		− ☐ ☐ +	
11:00 a.m.		− ☐ ☐ +	
12:00 p.m.		− ☐ ☐ +	
1:00 p.m.		− ☐ ☐ +	
2:00 p.m.		− ☐ ☐ +	
3:00 p.m.		− ☐ ☐ +	
4:00 p.m.		− ☐ ☐ +	
5:00 p.m.		− ☐ ☐ +	
6:00 p.m.		− ☐ ☐ +	
7:00 p.m.		− ☐ ☐ +	
8:00 p.m.		− ☐ ☐ +	
9:00 p.m.		− ☐ ☐ +	
10:00 p.m.		− ☐ ☐ +	

TIME	ACTIVITY	PRODUCTIVITY	MOOD TRACKER
6:00 a.m.		− ☐ ☐ +	
7:00 a.m.		− ☐ ☐ +	
8:00 a.m.		− ☐ ☐ +	
9:00 a.m.		− ☐ ☐ +	
10:00 a.m.		− ☐ ☐ +	
11:00 a.m.		− ☐ ☐ +	
12:00 p.m.		− ☐ ☐ +	
1:00 p.m.		− ☐ ☐ +	
2:00 p.m.		− ☐ ☐ +	
3:00 p.m.		− ☐ ☐ +	
4:00 p.m.		− ☐ ☐ +	
5:00 p.m.		− ☐ ☐ +	
6:00 p.m.		− ☐ ☐ +	
7:00 p.m.		− ☐ ☐ +	
8:00 p.m.		− ☐ ☐ +	
9:00 p.m.		− ☐ ☐ +	
10:00 p.m.		− ☐ ☐ +	

Blocking Out Your Time

Date	Month	Year

1. Make a list of things you want to complete in one given day in the TO DO column.

2. Order that list based on priority (the first thing on the list should be the most important).

3. Schedule the most important priorities for the first day and plan to complete them during your high-energy period. Fill in the rest of your TO DO list in the open spots in your day. Make sure to schedule in breaks and self care and match priority level with your energy level.

TIME	SCHEDULE	TO DO
8:00 a.m.		
9:00 a.m.		
10:00 a.m.		
11:00 a.m.		
12:00 p.m.		
1:00 p.m.		
2:00 p.m.		
3:00 p.m.		
4:00 p.m.		
5:00 p.m.		
6:00 p.m.		
7:00 p.m.		
8:00 p.m.		
9:00 p.m.		

	Date		Month		Year

TIME	SCHEDULE	TO DO
6:00 a.m.		
7:00 a.m.		
8:00 a.m.		
9:00 a.m.		
10:00 a.m.		
11:00 a.m.		
12:00 p.m.		
1:00 p.m.		
2:00 p.m.		
3:00 p.m.		
4:00 p.m.		
5:00 p.m.		
6:00 p.m.		
7:00 p.m.		
8:00 p.m.		
9:00 p.m.		
10:00 p.m.		

BLOCKING OUT YOUR TIME

Date	Month	Year

TIME	SCHEDULE	TO DO
6:00 a.m.		
7:00 a.m.		
8:00 a.m.		
9:00 a.m.		
10:00 a.m.		
11:00 a.m.		
12:00 p.m.		
1:00 p.m.		
2:00 p.m.		
3:00 p.m.		
4:00 p.m.		
5:00 p.m.		
6:00 p.m.		
7:00 p.m.		
8:00 p.m.		
9:00 p.m.		
10:00 p.m.		

Date   Month   Year

TIME	SCHEDULE	TO DO
6:00 a.m.		
7:00 a.m.		
8:00 a.m.		
9:00 a.m.		
10:00 a.m.		
11:00 a.m.		
12:00 p.m.		
1:00 p.m.		
2:00 p.m.		
3:00 p.m.		
4:00 p.m.		
5:00 p.m.		
6:00 p.m.		
7:00 p.m.		
8:00 p.m.		
9:00 p.m.		
10:00 p.m.		

BLOCKING OUT YOUR TIME

Date	Month	Year

TIME	SCHEDULE	TO DO
6:00 a.m.		
7:00 a.m.		
8:00 a.m.		
9:00 a.m.		
10:00 a.m.		
11:00 a.m.		
12:00 p.m.		
1:00 p.m.		
2:00 p.m.		
3:00 p.m.		
4:00 p.m.		
5:00 p.m.		
6:00 p.m.		
7:00 p.m.		
8:00 p.m.		
9:00 p.m.		
10:00 p.m.		

	Date	Month	Year

TIME	SCHEDULE	TO DO
6:00 a.m.		
7:00 a.m.		
8:00 a.m.		
9:00 a.m.		
10:00 a.m.		
11:00 a.m.		
12:00 p.m.		
1:00 p.m.		
2:00 p.m.		
3:00 p.m.		
4:00 p.m.		
5:00 p.m.		
6:00 p.m.		
7:00 p.m.		
8:00 p.m.		
9:00 p.m.		
10:00 p.m.		

BLOCKING OUT YOUR TIME

Date	Month	Year

TIME	SCHEDULE	TO DO
6:00 a.m.		
7:00 a.m.		
8:00 a.m.		
9:00 a.m.		
10:00 a.m.		
11:00 a.m.		
12:00 p.m.		
1:00 p.m.		
2:00 p.m.		
3:00 p.m.		
4:00 p.m.		
5:00 p.m.		
6:00 p.m.		
7:00 p.m.		
8:00 p.m.		
9:00 p.m.		
10:00 p.m.		

Date	Month	Year

TIME	SCHEDULE	TO DO
6:00 a.m.		
7:00 a.m.		
8:00 a.m.		
9:00 a.m.		
10:00 a.m.		
11:00 a.m.		
12:00 p.m.		
1:00 p.m.		
2:00 p.m.		
3:00 p.m.		
4:00 p.m.		
5:00 p.m.		
6:00 p.m.		
7:00 p.m.		
8:00 p.m.		
9:00 p.m.		
10:00 p.m.		

BLOCKING OUT YOUR TIME

Date	Month	Year

TIME	SCHEDULE	TO DO
6:00 a.m.		
7:00 a.m.		
8:00 a.m.		
9:00 a.m.		
10:00 a.m.		
11:00 a.m.		
12:00 p.m.		
1:00 p.m.		
2:00 p.m.		
3:00 p.m.		
4:00 p.m.		
5:00 p.m.		
6:00 p.m.		
7:00 p.m.		
8:00 p.m.		
9:00 p.m.		
10:00 p.m.		

	Date	Month	Year

TIME	SCHEDULE	TO DO
6:00 a.m.		
7:00 a.m.		
8:00 a.m.		
9:00 a.m.		
10:00 a.m.		
11:00 a.m.		
12:00 p.m.		
1:00 p.m.		
2:00 p.m.		
3:00 p.m.		
4:00 p.m.		
5:00 p.m.		
6:00 p.m.		
7:00 p.m.		
8:00 p.m.		
9:00 p.m.		
10:00 p.m.		

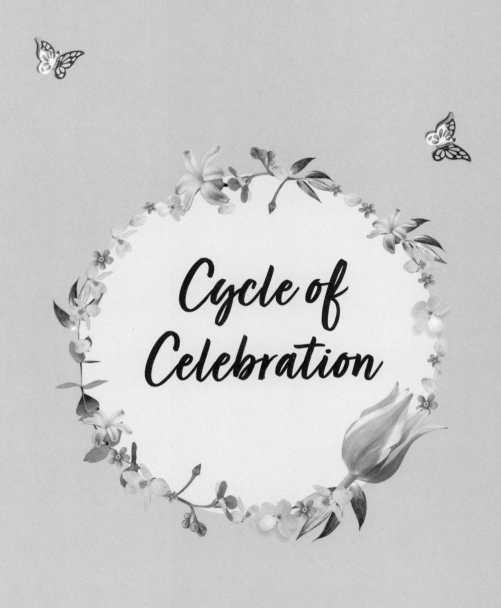

Cycle of
Celebration

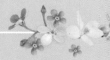

I n our fast-paced, achievement-based society, it's easy to get caught in a cycle: set a goal, achieve the goal, and then immediately set another goal. Being motivated is wonderful, but if you don't acknowledge and celebrate your achievements, you could be heading for burnout.

The goal-achievement-goal cycle above is missing two steps: fascination and celebration.

Fascination can be reawakened by trying novel things without attachment to the outcome. It can be difficult to remove outcome attachment because it is normal for your inner critic and perfectionist to show up and ruin the moment by telling you that whatever you're trying, doing, or creating "isn't good enough." The beautiful thing about being a child is that the outcome doesn't matter—it's the doing that provides joy.

Celebration allows you to really enjoy the steps you took achieve your goal and rewards this behavior in such a way that encourages it to be repeated over and over again.

This cycle allows you to keep moving forward in life, growing, and progressing. But it also encourages you to enjoy the fruits of your labor, stay present, feel a sense of pride in your achievements (you deserve to feel good about the things you accomplish!), and recharge before tackling the next goal.

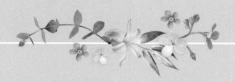

Exercise in Fascination

Remove "perfection" from your vocabulary. Your inner perfectionist and its chronic fear of failure will sabotage your chances at happiness.

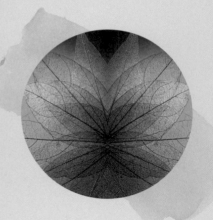

Try incorporating the following activities into your life to silence the inner "perfectionist," a.k.a. your happiness saboteur. Once you've silenced your inner perfectionist, you can move on to the next step of becoming fascinated with things.

List some fun things that you're curious about that you've never tried or explored before. Let the list get wild, and then put stars next to your favorites to help narrow down your goal.

Set a Goal

Use your manifestation techniques to outline what your goal will look like. Highlight the subtle differences in your life as you achieve this. Write your goal at the bottom of the page and then list every conceivable facet of change you think will have to happen to get you in the right mindset.

Achieve Your Goal

Break your goal into three slightly smaller goals. And then break those goals into smaller segments. By chunking your goals into smaller and easier-to-obtain steps, you can ride each little dopamine rush into the next one. Start with your goal and break each big step into slightly smaller steps.

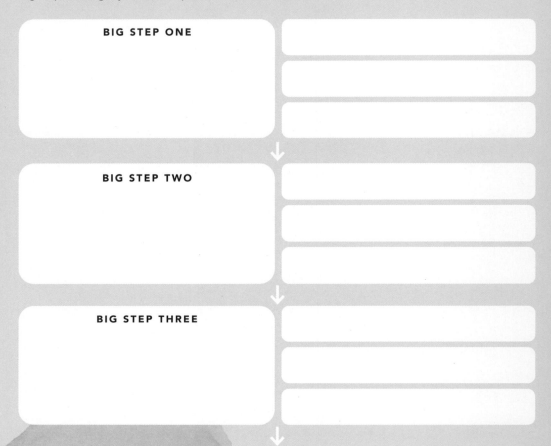

BIG STEP ONE

BIG STEP TWO

BIG STEP THREE

GOAL

Celebrate Your Success

The way you celebrate is entirely up to you, because different things feel good for different people. Draft up a list of possible celebrations prior to beginning work on your goal. If your goals are bigger than most, each step should have it's own appropriate award. Do anything your heart desires. The important thing is that you recognize you're rejoicing something that you have not only earned, but rightly deserve.

Once you've celebrated your success, you can happily move on to the next goal!

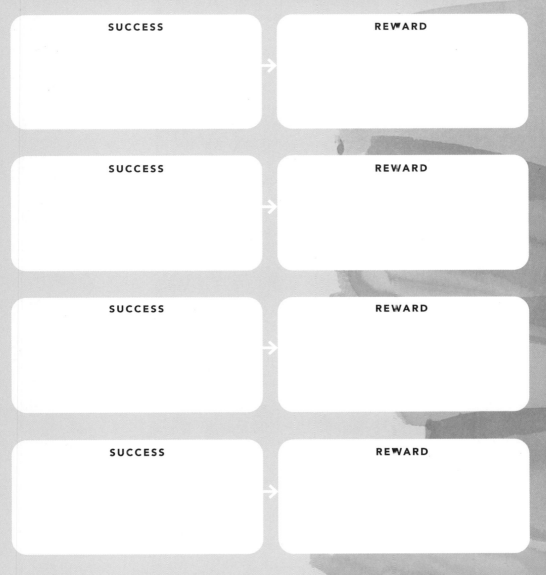

SUCCESS		REWARD
	→	
SUCCESS		REWARD
	→	
SUCCESS		REWARD
	→	
SUCCESS		REWARD
	→	

Exercise in Fascination

Remove "perfection" from your vocabulary. Your inner perfectionist and its chronic fear of failure will sabotage your chances at happiness.

Try incorporating the following activities into your life to silence the inner "perfectionist," a.k.a. your happiness saboteur. Once you've silenced your inner perfectionist, you can move on to the next step of becoming fascinated with things.

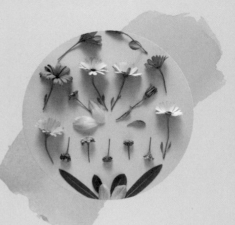

List some fun things that you're curious about that you've never tried or explored before. Let the list get wild, and then put stars next to your favorites to help narrow down your goal.

Set a Goal

Use your manifestation techniques to outline what your goal will look like. Highlight the subtle differences in your life as you achieve this. Write your goal at the bottom of the page and then list every conceivable facet of change you think will have to happen to get you in the right mindset.

Achieve Your Goal

Break your goal into three slightly smaller goals. And then break those goals into smaller segments. By chunking your goals into smaller and easier-to-obtain steps, you can ride each little dopamine rush into the next one. Start with your goal and break each big step into slightly smaller steps.

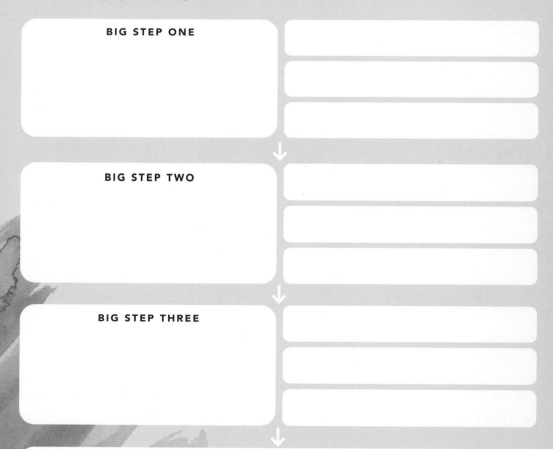

BIG STEP ONE

BIG STEP TWO

BIG STEP THREE

GOAL

Celebrate Your Success

The way you celebrate is entirely up to you, because different things feel good for different people. Draft up a list of possible celebrations prior to beginning work on your goal. If your goals are bigger than most, each step should have it's own appropriate award. Do anything your heart desires. The important thing is that you recognize you're rejoicing something that you have not only earned, but rightly deserve.

Once you've celebrated your success, you can happily move on to the next goal!

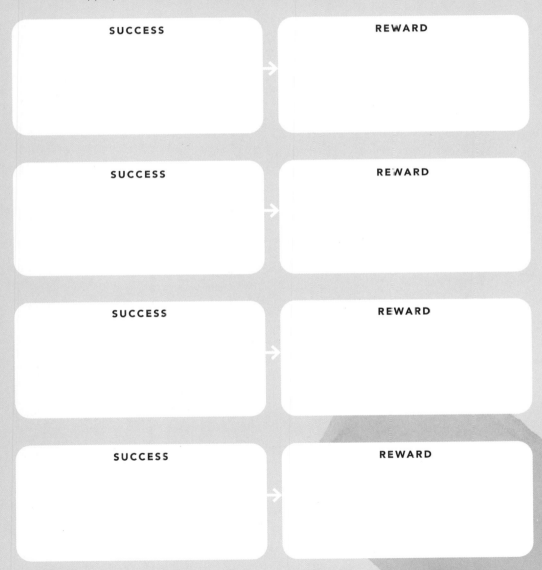

SUCCESS

REWARD

SUCCESS

REWARD

SUCCESS

REWARD

SUCCESS

REWARD

Exercise in Fascination

Remove "perfection" from your vocabulary.
Your inner perfectionist and its chronic fear of
failure will sabotage your chances at happiness.

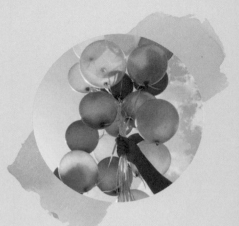

Try incorporating the following activities into
your life to silence the inner "perfectionist,"
a.k.a. your happiness saboteur. Once you've
silenced your inner perfectionist, you can move
on to the next step of becoming fascinated
with things.

List some fun things that you're curious about that you've never tried or explored before.
Let the list get wild, and then put stars next to your favorites to help narrow down your goal.

Set a Goal

Use your manifestation techniques to outline what your goal will look like. Highlight the subtle differences in your life as you achieve this. Write your goal at the bottom of the page and then list every conceivable facet of change you think will have to happen to get you in the right mindset.

Achieve Your Goal

Break your goal into three slightly smaller goals. And then break those goals into smaller segments. By chunking your goals into smaller and easier-to-obtain steps, you can ride each little dopamine rush into the next one. Start with your goal and break each big step into slightly smaller steps.

BIG STEP ONE

BIG STEP TWO

BIG STEP THREE

GOAL

Celebrate Your Success

The way you celebrate is entirely up to you, because different things feel good for different people. Draft up a list of possible celebrations prior to beginning work on your goal. If your goals are bigger than most, each step should have it's own appropriate award. Do anything your heart desires. The important thing is that you recognize you're rejoicing something that you have not only earned, but rightly deserve.

Once you've celebrated your success, you can happily move on to the next goal!

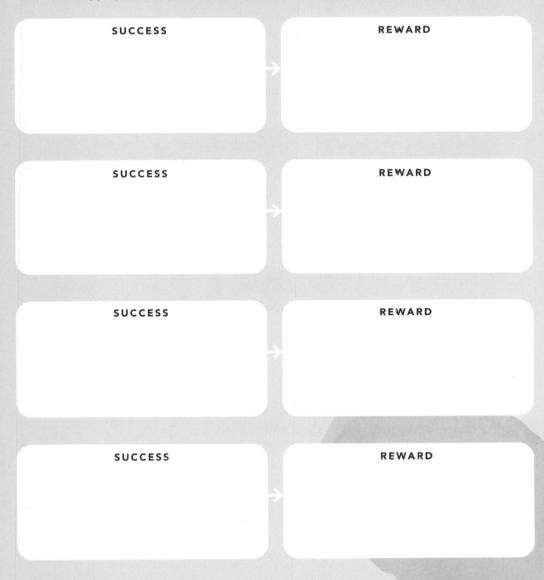

SUCCESS

REWARD

SUCCESS

REWARD

SUCCESS

REWARD

SUCCESS

REWARD

Exercise in Fascination

Remove "perfection" from your vocabulary. Your inner perfectionist and its chronic fear of failure will sabotage your chances at happiness.

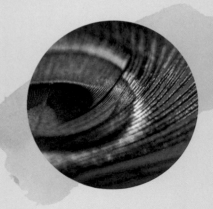

Try incorporating the following activities into your life to silence the inner "perfectionist," a.k.a. your happiness saboteur. Once you've silenced your inner perfectionist, you can move on to the next step of becoming fascinated with things.

List some fun things that you're curious about that you've never tried or explored before. Let the list get wild, and then put stars next to your favorites to help narrow down your goal.

Set a Goal

Use your manifestation techniques to outline what your goal will look like. Highlight the subtle differences in your life as you achieve this. Write your goal at the bottom of the page and then list every conceivable facet of change you think will have to happen to get you in the right mindset.

Achieve Your Goal

Break your goal into three slightly smaller goals. And then break those goals into smaller segments. By chunking your goals into smaller and easier-to-obtain steps, you can ride each little dopamine rush into the next one. Start with your goal and break each big step into slightly smaller steps.

BIG STEP ONE

BIG STEP TWO

BIG STEP THREE

GOAL

Celebrate Your Success

The way you celebrate is entirely up to you, because different things feel good for different people. Draft up a list of possible celebrations prior to beginning work on your goal. If your goals are bigger than most, each step should have it's own appropriate award. Do anything your heart desires. The important thing is that you recognize you're rejoicing something that you have not only earned, but rightly deserve.

Once you've celebrated your success, you can happily move on to the next goal!

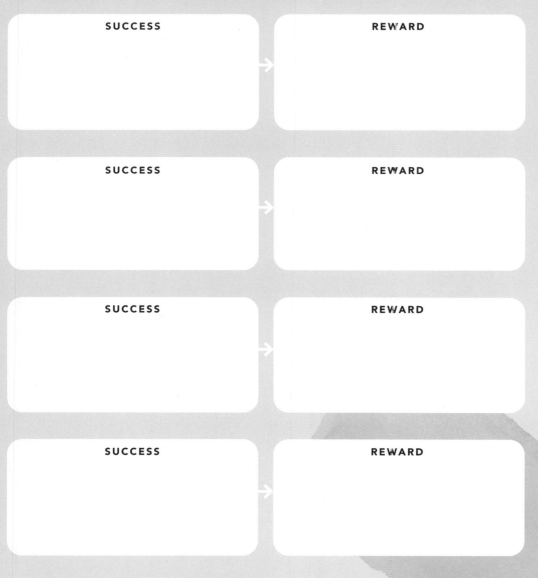

SUCCESS → **REWARD**

SUCCESS → **REWARD**

SUCCESS → **REWARD**

SUCCESS → **REWARD**

Exercise in Fascination

Remove "perfection" from your vocabulary. Your inner perfectionist and its chronic fear of failure will sabotage your chances at happiness.

Try incorporating the following activities into your life to silence the inner "perfectionist," a.k.a. your happiness saboteur. Once you've silenced your inner perfectionist, you can move on to the next step of becoming fascinated with things.

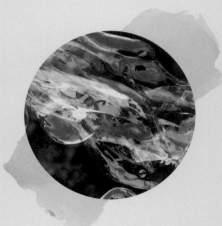

List some fun things that you're curious about that you've never tried or explored before. Let the list get wild, and then put stars next to your favorites to help narrow down your goal.

Set a Goal

Use your manifestation techniques to outline what your goal will look like. Highlight the subtle differences in your life as you achieve this. Write your goal at the bottom of the page and then list every conceivable facet of change you think will have to happen to get you in the right mindset.

Achieve Your Goal

Break your goal into three slightly smaller goals. And then break those goals into smaller segments. By chunking your goals into smaller and easier-to-obtain steps, you can ride each little dopamine rush into the next one. Start with your goal and break each big step into slightly smaller steps.

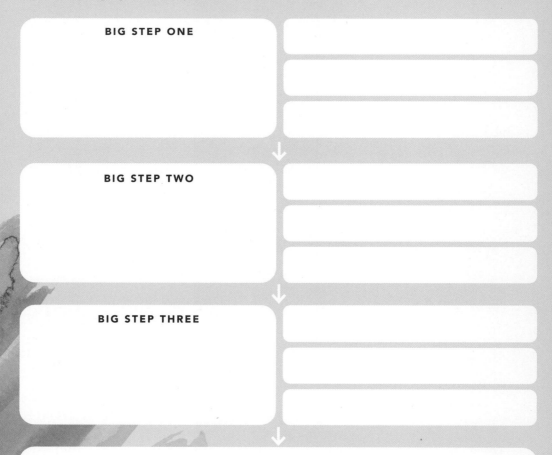

BIG STEP ONE

BIG STEP TWO

BIG STEP THREE

GOAL

Celebrate Your Success

The way you celebrate is entirely up to you, because different things feel good for different people. Draft up a list of possible celebrations prior to beginning work on your goal. If your goals are bigger than most, each step should have it's own appropriate award. Do anything your heart desires. The important thing is that you recognize you're rejoicing something that you have not only earned, but rightly deserve.

Once you've celebrated your success, you can happily move on to the next goal!

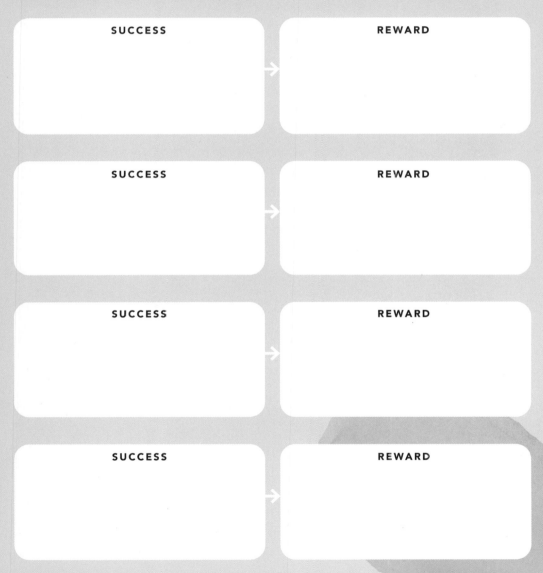

SUCCESS

REWARD

SUCCESS

REWARD

SUCCESS

REWARD

SUCCESS

REWARD

Exercise in Fascination

Remove "perfection" from your vocabulary. Your inner perfectionist and its chronic fear of failure will sabotage your chances at happiness.

Try incorporating the following activities into your life to silence the inner "perfectionist," a.k.a. your happiness saboteur. Once you've silenced your inner perfectionist, you can move on to the next step of becoming fascinated with things.

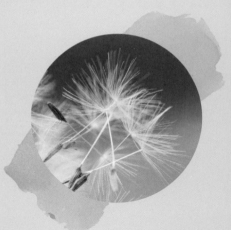

List some fun things that you're curious about that you've never tried or explored before. Let the list get wild, and then put stars next to your favorites to help narrow down your goal.

Set a Goal

Use your manifestation techniques to outline what your goal will look like. Highlight the subtle differences in your life as you achieve this. Write your goal at the bottom of the page and then list every conceivable facet of change you think will have to happen to get you in the right mindset.

Achieve Your Goal

Break your goal into three slightly smaller goals. And then break those goals into smaller segments. By chunking your goals into smaller and easier-to-obtain steps, you can ride each little dopamine rush into the next one. Start with your goal and break each big step into slightly smaller steps.

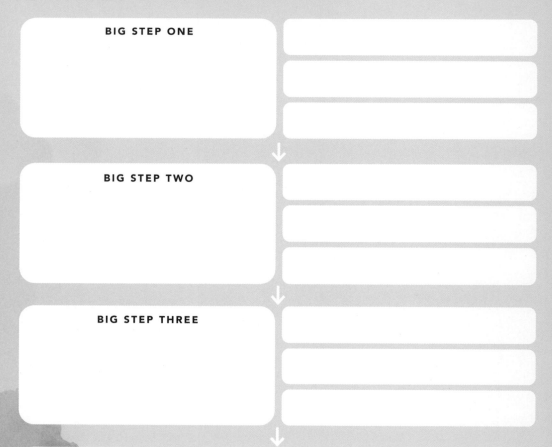

BIG STEP ONE

BIG STEP TWO

BIG STEP THREE

GOAL

Celebrate Your Success

The way you celebrate is entirely up to you, because different things feel good for different people. Draft up a list of possible celebrations prior to beginning work on your goal. If your goals are bigger than most, each step should have it's own appropriate award. Do anything your heart desires. The important thing is that you recognize you're rejoicing something that you have not only earned, but rightly deserve.

Once you've celebrated your success, you can happily move on to the next goal!

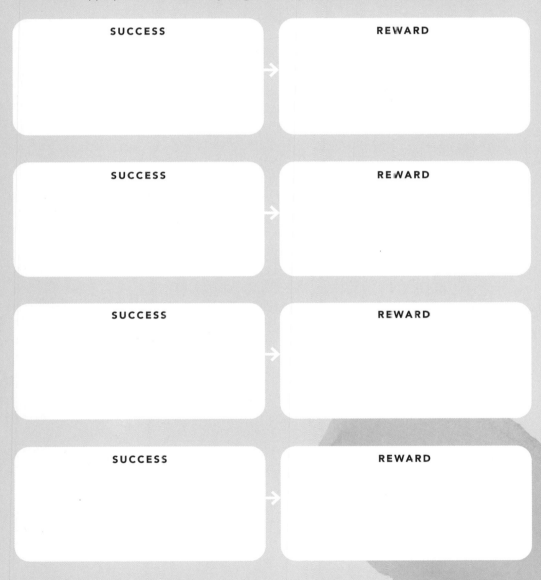

SUCCESS → **REWARD**

SUCCESS → **REWARD**

SUCCESS → **REWARD**

SUCCESS → **REWARD**

Self Love

Do you love yourself? Do you show yourself empathy, kindness, and understanding? Do you find yourself thrilling, exciting, astonishing, and captivating? This type of self-love comes first—love yourself and the rest will follow. There's only one definition of love that truly matters: the one you define within yourself. To figure this out, you have to do the work. You have to take a deep dive into who you are and relentlessly pursue yourself with a fervent passion.

If you're like most people, you probably don't love yourself completely yet. But good news: this kind of love can be learned. Even better news: self-love is the ultimate form of self-care. When you learn how to love yourself, it becomes easier to attract the right kind of love (platonic and romantic) into your life. You can then set clear boundaries (because you know your worth), love someone else without being co-dependent, make decisions that align with who you are, and achieve internal emotional stability.

Self-love might sound like a radical concept, but it's not. It simply takes the love, attention, affection, forgiveness, happiness, acceptance, and joy that you give to others, and turns it inward before sharing your love with others.

How do you learn to love yourself? The activities in this section will help you achieve an everlasting self-love. And, if the love you have for yourself should ever waver, simply repeat these exercises at any time to reignite the spark.

Gratitude Journal

One of the best things you can do for your mindset is to adopt an attitude of gratitude. Learning to be grateful for the smallest things is one of the quickest ways to have a happy life. Sometimes it can be hard to see the good things in your life, especially when overwhelm, exhaustion, or emotional pain enter the picture.

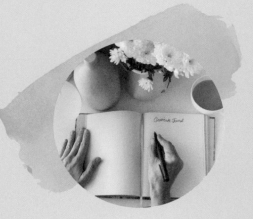

In these moments of pain, it is especially important to have a list of things you're grateful for. You can reread them as a reminder of all of the good that does exist—even when the bad clouds your ability to see it.

Starting a gratitude journal is an amazing way to guarantee that you'll always have something to read—a book of your own creation—that can lift your spirits.

Add one thing that you're grateful for at the end of every day. Once this is filled up, you'll have a year's worth of gratitude to look back on and remember fondly.

1

2

3

4

5

6

7

8

9

10

11

12

13

14

15

16

17

18

19

20

21

22

23

24

25

26

27

28

29

30

31

32

33

34

35

36

37

38

39

40

41

42

43

44

45

46

47

48

49

50

51

52

53

54

55

56

57

58

59

60

61

62

63

64

65

66

67

68

69

70

71

72

73

74

75

76

77

78

79

80

81

82

83

84

85

86

87

88

89

90

91

92

93

94

95

96

97

98

99

100

101

102

103

104

105

106

107

108

109

110

111

112

113

114

115

116

117

118

119

120

121

122

123

124

125

126

127

128

129

130

131

132

133

134

135

136

137

138

139

140

141

142

143

144

145

146

147

148

149

150

151

152

153

154

155

156

157

158

159

160

161

162

163

164

165

166

167

168

169

170

171

172

173

174

175

176

177

178

179

180

181

182

183

184

185

186

187

188

189

190

191

192

193

194

195

196

197

198

199

200

201

202

203

204

205

206

207

208

209

210

211

212

213

214

215

216

217

218

219

220

221

222

223

224

225

226

227

228

229

230

231

232

233

234

235

236

237

238

239

240

241

242

243

244

245

246

247

248

249

250

251

252

253

254

255

256

257

258

259

260

261

262

263

264

265

266

267

268

269

270

271

272

273

274

275

276

277

278

279

280

281

282

283

284

285

286

287

288

289

290

291

292

293

294

295

296

297

298

299

300

301

302

303

304

305

306

307

308

309

310

311

312

313

314

315

316

317

318

319

320

321

322

323

324

325

326

327

328

329

330

331

332

333

334

335

336

337

338

339

340

341

342

343

344

345

346

347

348

349

350

351

352

353

354

355

356

357

358

359

360

361

362

363

364

365

Flip the Script

Sometimes our intrusive and patently untrue thoughts are the loudest and the ones that we listen to. If this happens to you, try to flip the script. Take an **original thought** with a not-so-nice intent, and then challenge that thought.

Re-frame it with a positive spin, so that you're no longer torturing yourself with your own thoughts. Once you've filled up these pages, you can cut the dotted line and only be left with the positive **challenge thoughts** and interpretations.

ORIGINAL THOUGHT

CHALLENGE THOUGHT

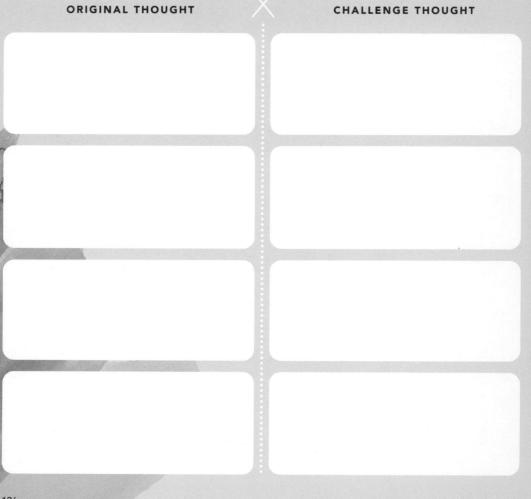

ORIGINAL THOUGHT

CHALLENGE THOUGHT

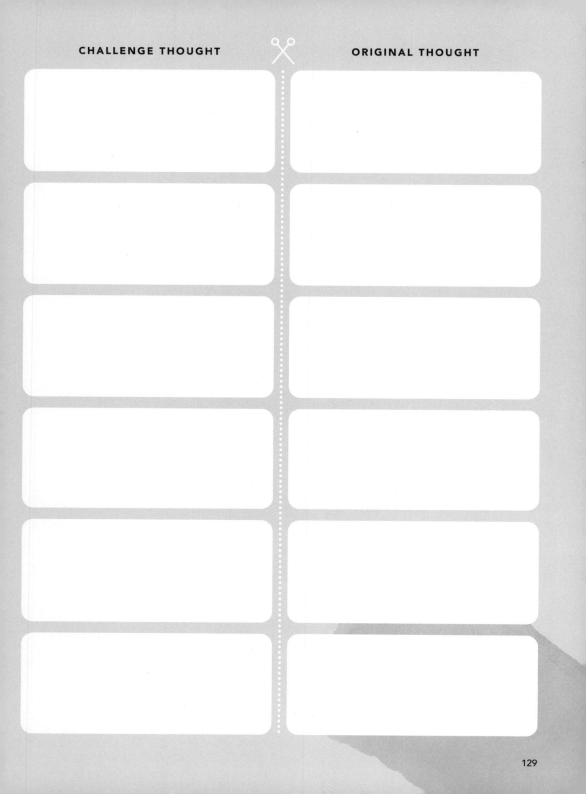

ORIGINAL THOUGHT   CHALLENGE THOUGHT

ORIGINAL THOUGHT ✂ CHALLENGE THOUGHT

Replacing Negative Thoughts with Positive Ones

This exercise is very similar to the previous one. In **negative self-talk** column, make a list of the things you either don't like about yourself or think you need to change about yourself. This part of the exercise may be a bit painful, but it's necessary to identify your pain points so you can resolve the issues surrounding them.

Now you can begin to rewire your thinking. In the right column, write a positive **affirmation** that counters the negative self-talk. Think of it like an argument: your brain is telling you one thing, and now you're going to tell your brain that it must be mistaken.

Some negative thoughts might be more difficult to get rid of, and need multiple affirmations. Feel free to enter in your negative self-talk more than once to try and inspire positive affirmations that hit all the right points.

NEGATIVE SELF-TALK ✂ AFFIRMATION

AFFIRMATION

✂

NEGATIVE SELF-TALK

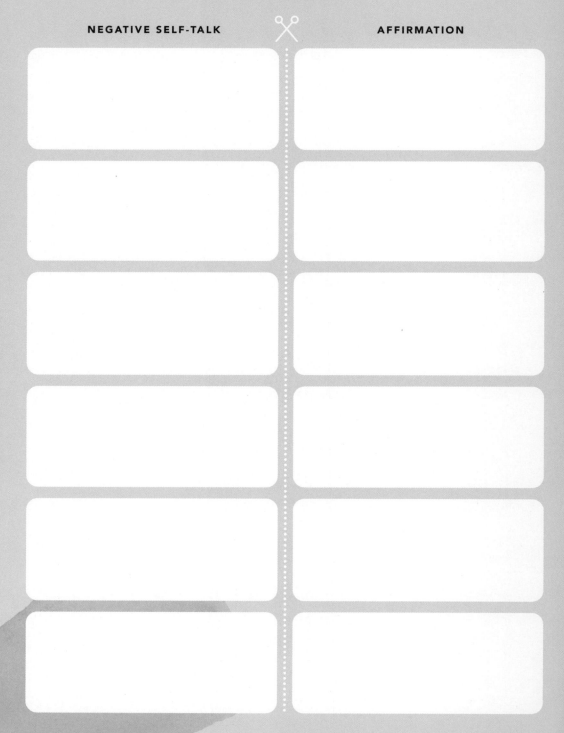

NEGATIVE SELF-TALK

AFFIRMATION

NEGATIVE SELF-TALK

AFFIRMATION

AFFIRMATION | **NEGATIVE SELF-TALK**

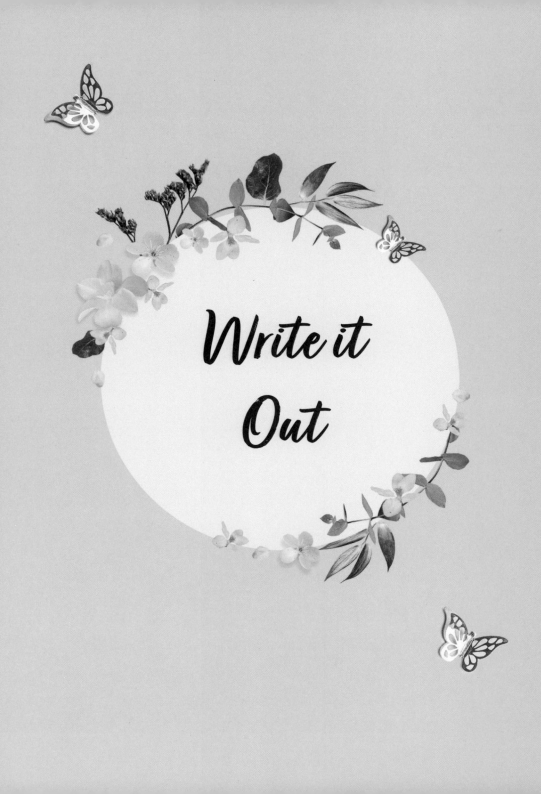

Write it
Out

Writing is an excellent way to get out of your own head. Writing letters to yourself helps you remove yourself from your own inhibitions and create a life that is full to the brim with things you want to enjoy.

Living in the past—where regret, second-guessing, loss, grief, and painful memories exist—can cause you to feel depressed. Living in the future—where fear, confusion, control issues, unknowns, and a series of "what-ifs" exist—can cause you to feel anxious. Getting you to a place where you can embrace the present moment will increase your awareness, gratitude, and self-love, which are all components of self care. The following exercises involve writing letters to yourself as a way to clear your internal blocks and make way for love.

For those days when writing letters to yourself just seems like too much mental effort, you can respond to one of the journal prompts instead to get your creative juices flowing and to unblock yourself.

These prompts are effective because they shift your mind to a place of imagination and hope and force you to employ gratitude and optimism. The prompts also put you in a place where you must remove your self-limiting beliefs. The more you practice forcing your mindset to shift in this way the easier it will be to shift your mood on your own.

Letter to Your Past Self

Write yourself a letter addressing things that have happened in the past. Be patient and gentle with yourself during this process. There are no rules for what you can write about—the only requisite is that you write about things that happened in the past.

It's normal if you find this writing exercise emotionally exhausting. Sometimes self-care involves the acknowledgment of painful moments to help you fully release them.

Date	Month	Year

Dear _____

_____

_____

_____

_____

_____

_____

_____

_____

_____

Letter to Your Future Self

Without any external distractions, use the thin black marker to write a letter about your hopes, dreams, and even your fears. The only rule here is that everything you write about needs to be hypothetical and in the future—there should be nothing in this letter that has already come to fruition. Write candidly and openly.

Allow yourself to explore your dreams and fears freely. When you're done writing, take the thick black marker and cross off any fears you wrote down: this sends a signal to your mind that these fears are gone. Now you're only going to put thought and intention toward achieving your dreams.

Date	Month	Year

Dear _____

_____

_____

_____

_____

_____

_____

_____

_____

Love Letter to Yourself

Write yourself a madly passionate love letter. Praise yourself. Pretend that you're the one true love of your life (spoiler: you should be). Focus on things that make you beautiful (physically, mentally, and emotionally), your unique qualities, your remarkable traits, or things you just really like/love about yourself. When you're done writing, re-read it every day until your loving thoughts about yourself become who you truly are.

Date	Month	Year

Dear _____

_____

_____

_____

_____

_____

_____

_____

_____

Dialogue with Yourself

1. What's your perfect day? Describe it in detail from morning to night.

2. Write a tribute to your favorite person and pretend it will be read aloud at an awards show held in his or her honor.

_____

_____

_____

_____

_____

_____

_____

_____

_____

_____

_____

_____

_____

_____

_____

3. A genie appears and grants you three wishes. What are they? Why did you wish for these things?

4. You've just won $100 million and have seven days to spend it!
Write the story of what happens during those seven days.

5. A knock is at your door—it's a reality television show offering to build your dream house! They need to know where you want it built and what you want it to look like. What do you say?

_____

_____

_____

_____

_____

_____

_____

_____

_____

_____

_____

_____

_____

_____

_____

_____

6. You have ten minutes to meet with the President of the United States. What you say in those ten minutes will greatly influence the President and the course of history. What do you say?

7. You get to have dinner with anyone who has ever existed, living or dead. Who do you choose? What do you eat? What do you discuss?

_____

_____

_____

_____

_____

_____

_____

_____

_____

_____

_____

_____

_____

_____

_____

8. You have a time machine and can only use it once. What time period do you choose and why?

9. You can go back as an adult to visit yourself as a child. What age do you revisit? Why? What advice or guidance do you give yourself, if any?

10. You die at the age of one hundred. What does your obituary say?

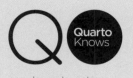

Inspiring | Educating | Creating | Entertaining

Brimming with creative inspiration, how-to projects, and useful information to enrich your everyday life, Quarto Knows is a favorite destination for those pursuing their interests and passions. Visit our site and dig deeper with our books into your area of interest: Quarto Creates, Quarto Cooks, Quarto Homes, Quarto Lives, Quarto Drives, Quarto Explores, Quarto Gifts, or Quarto Kids.

First published in 2021 by Chartwell Books, an imprint of The Quarto Group, 142 West 36th Street, 4th Floor, New York, NY 10018, USA
T (212) 779-4972 F (212) 779-6058
www.QuartoKnows.com

Contains content originally published in 2020 as *The Complete Guide to Self Care* by Chartwell Books, an imprint of The Quarto Group, 142 West 36th Street, 4th Floor, New York, NY, 10018.

Chartwell titles are also available at discount for retail, wholesale, promotional, and bulk purchase. For details, contact the Special Sales Manager by email at specialsales@quarto.com or by mail at The Quarto Group, Attn: Special Sales Manager, 100 Cummings Center Suite 265D, Beverly, MA 01915 USA.

10 9 8 7 6 5 4 3

ISBN: 978-0-7858-3924-8

Publisher: Rage Kindelsperger
Creative Director: Laura Drew
Managing Editor: Cara Donaldson
Project Editor: Leeann Moreau
Cover and Interior Design: Evelin Kasikov

Printed in China

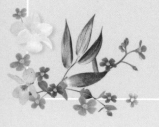

This journal provides general information on various widely known and widely accepted topics in the area of self-care and wellness. However, it should not be relied upon as recommending or promoting any specific diagnosis or method of treatment for a particular condition, and it is not intended as a substitute for medical advice or for direct diagnosis and treatment of a medical condition by a qualified physician. Readers who have questions about a particular condition, possible treatments for that condition, or possible reactions from the condition or its treatment should consult a physician or other qualified healthcare professional.